THE UPCYCLED HEALING BRAIN

Luca M Damiani is an artist, author and university fellow, focusing his ongoing creative practice and research on neuroscience/ health, technology and nature. His work also crosses over with human rights and social design.

Luca has a neurological disability and has had various books of visual art and academic articles published, as well as his art exhibited internationally. He has worked and collaborated with institutions such as BMJ Medical Humanities, Mozilla, Amnesty International, BBC, Science Gallery, Computer Arts Society, Disney, University of the Arts London, Yale University, Jewish Book Council, The Times of Israel, TATE, V&A and more.

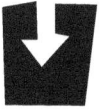

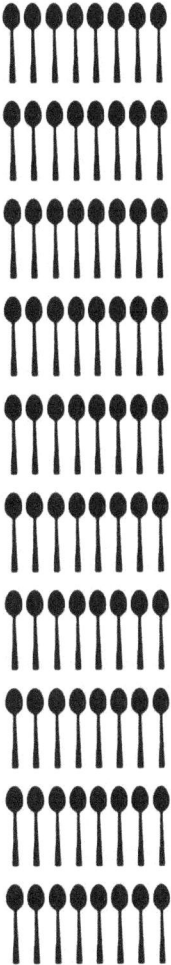

THE UPCYCLED HEALING BRAIN

An Eco-Therapy Diary in 80 buried spoons

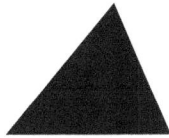

Luca M Damiani

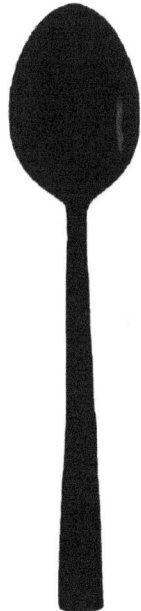

VP

First published in 2024 by Valley Press
Woodend, The Crescent, Scarborough, UK, YO11 2PW
www.valleypressuk.com

ISBN 978-1-915606-39-6
Cat. no. VP0236

To my Ls

Introduction

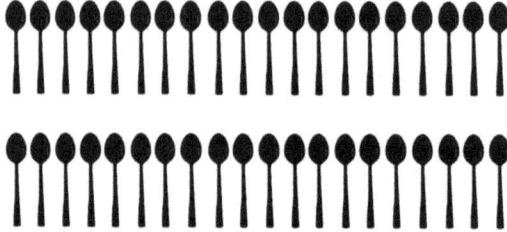

The Upcycled Healing Brain is a diary, a hybrid memoir. It reflects my lived experience of neurological and sensory disability. I am assessed with a 52% impairment of my central nervous system (CNS) function, and this was due to an accident in January 2018 which caused me a neurological trauma, having a life changing impact. The CNS is a complex functional system, and the trauma has triggered a combination of different neurological conditions causing stimuli overloads, sensory sensitivities, chronic pain and fatigue, short memory loss, daily vertigo attacks, persistent dizziness, brain overloads, brain fog, hallucinations and dissociations. It also changed the chemicals' flow in my brain, hence also triggering various mental health conditions. All this also has cross-reacted and formed various brain meltdowns in connection to my high-functioning autism. So, it has been a complex journey to adapt to for me, for my family, for my loves and for my friends.

In a long (and ongoing) journey of rehabilitation, there were times spent in mental health unit, times of self-harming due to pain and sensory overloads, times of suicidal ideation (and sadly one attempt) and times of loss. There has been an ongoing acceptance of living with a life changing invisible disability that affects my normal daily functioning; there is a constant new self discovery, and this book has been a huge part of forming a positive angle of who I am and who I can be. I have decided to share this journey because other memoirs from people who have experienced trauma have helped me to partly understand and process mine, becoming an important part of my recovery and acceptance. And so, I hope that my story can help others' too. One day. Maybe.

Why the title *The Upcycled Healing Brain: An Eco-Therapy Diary in 80 Buried Spoons*? Because:

- The whole book has been created embedded in therapeutic settings in nature whilst healing.
- I have created the design-layout of the writing and the artworks in the book to reflect my diaries.
- Following the metaphor of a spoon as a limited quantity of daily energy in chronic illness (based on Spoon Theory), I explored my condition in spoons, as my energy and health allowed me to.
- I love traveling, but haven't been able to travel since 2018 due to my disability - and so I felt like engaging in an imaginary journey with 80 spoons of energy (like Phileas Fogg!) in my own brain.
- All my 80 spoons (my poems and artworks/designs) were also buried and planted in nature, mainly in *The Upcycled Healing Garden* (an actual therapy garden) I have been designing in Markwick Gardens in St Leonards-on-Sea (Hastings, UK). I have buried all these 80 pieces there in order to feed new plants that are now growing strong.
- Hence, bringing life from a painful journey, with the meaning of "Upcycling" as a method for rebuilding my inner self and reconstructing it from something that was once broken.

I hope you will like this book and thank you very much for reading!

Luca xx

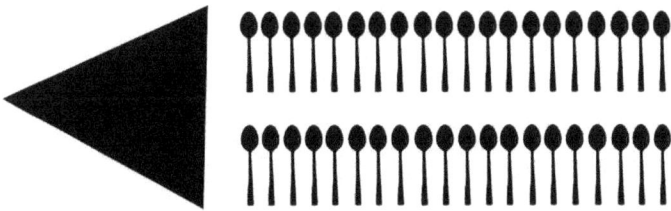

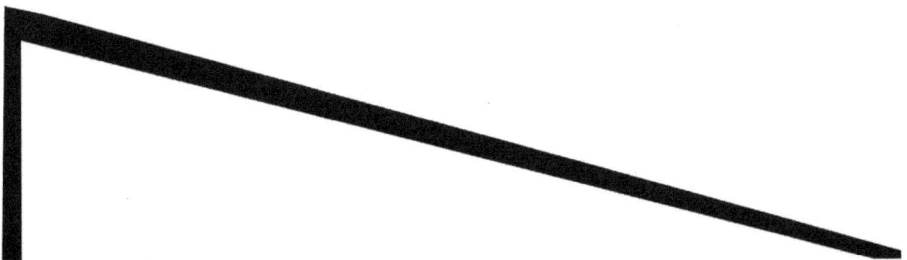

Spoon_01 : Bears (and idioms) in my Mind

One day, it was raining cats and dogs: it literally was.

As I looked up,
I had a bear on my head.

"Angel Cow!" - I thought, whilst taking a nurse by his evil horns
and weaseling the doctor out of the room.

Suddenly, as a fish out of water, I watched like a hawk
that hospital food : two birds, three bees and one blue pony.

That really got my "greatest of all time" nerve, and:

"Hold your horse shit!" - I shouted.
and let the food meow out of the plate.

What a wild chase then started, with clammed UP security,
and an eager gorilla making a block.
And so it was, 'Copycat,
quick cold fluid:
stars I could see, soft sounds I would do.
And I waited in blue calm lights
until sleep came home.

That is how I felt at times of my journey in neurological trauma.

Sometimes literally losing it and obsessing
about animal idioms to the point of melting down. It
has been a long and tough process of rehabilitation.

I am just writing this up after having met with my psychiatrist and I am now sitting on the beach looking at France in the horizon of this wonderful British sea-side coastal town. "Happy Now Here!" I think, staying still in the moment of this new year just staring up at the starred skies.

Spoon_02 : As The Spoon Empties

As the spoon empties,
it is difficult to walk.

As the spoon empties,
it is challenging to see.

As the spoon empties,
I am sorry for not functioning.

Chronic flow in sensory disability,
turning self into a spoonie,
damn those knives and forks!

Impaired central nervous system,
almost like a sudden crashed broken plate.

I wish I could have more spoons...
...maybe even teaspoons
as those could still help indeed.

The reality is that I only have the spoon I have today,
but I should be able to refill it tomorrow,
and that is what matters most.

Day by day,

spoon by spoon.

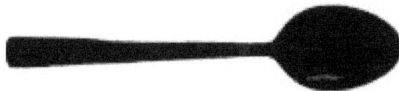

Spoon_03 : Shut Up - You must Talk

In the quiet flow of the hardest feeling, I stand and fall. In what? I don't really know. The feel of going backwards catches me in the spirit of saint lights and evil fire in my weakness. Scared of a lonely painful heart, I walk in **stillness** and embrace the rain. My steps of walking in cracking leaves are on **grounds** forgotten by the beasts. I am sleepy by the pill and I am awake by the "tinnie", and then I hear the voice on top of the tree: "Progress isn't always a straight line

and there will be challenges

and setbacks

along the way."

Space to grieve. Space to rebuild whatever is in **me**. Space to gain more self awareness. I leave the comfortable known, for a direction in the unknown. I am totally lost in this adventure.

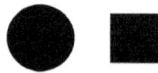

I feel my heart cracking sorrows.

In fragility I respond, **in** weakness I fight. I don't know what is to come, I don't know if I'll stand by. Day to day, focusing on the present moment of deep cuts, and the next step seems to be too far. In the details of daily wandering, I look for my balance and I look for you. I am **broken**, I surrender. Please give me the strength to rebuild from here.I do not have the answers nor I have a timeline, but stay with me and hold me, please. Resetting myself in processing identity, now a different being, I need to find who

I am. Who I can be. Memories connected to my deeper love and **essence**, are bringing me back to who I was, bringing pain in what was lost. In this new venture of existence, allowing space to reshape my soul, I stay in the present building trellis, for a new life to grow. Re-lived trauma, giving me a kick in my teeth, and punching me down to the floor, leaving me in a bloody lake.

I feel so very beaten-up today, in my heart and in my soul, with a drilling sound in my head. Can I rebuild? Can I rebuild not for who I was, but for who I am now and who I could be? I am sorry to bother you with this. "Shut up : You must talk", the wise red bear said.

And so in words I put it down.
Gotta go now, I have a long walk to do today.

Spoon_04 : 'Sea' You There

Suddenly walking with an unexpected real swinging feel of heart-beats' race. I was just gardening my soul...let me be! And yet, shining through the trees is the light of flowing particles, kinda lost, kinda clear, kinda hypothetical in their essence.

It is not the right time of day. Definitely it isn't, with all the broken tiles of inner being, currently in mosaic reconstruction: "Work in progress", the sign said.

Analyzing bit by bit in search of a pragmatic abstention for rational forced choice overtaking emotions.

But what does that even mean? I don't know. I am sure I should only be honest.

And so it comes, the steady answer clearly smashed. One, two, three or more channels of thoughtful reflections, shaping into blood circulation. So I hope.

Maybe.

At some point.

I am just worried when,

and perhaps you'll have stopped swimming.

Spoon_05 : In Stepping Words

As the day goes
in stepping words of whistling wind,
I am called by **you**r blue-tiful being.

In neurological trauma and disorder,
in this new invisible chronic pain of disability,
I lose my balance in my soul.

With steps of broken faith in who I am

I **move** away from the steady path.

It's not how it seems
in that smile covering deep pain,
and in that healthy body showing strength in its fragility.

It took a second to break down,
and it's taking a while to reconstruct.

But with these steps towards the almighty Rose, I try to look for what can be,
I try to accept a new way.
I know it is not as easy.
But slowly moving, we will get somewhere.

Anywhere.

Spoon_06 : My broken neurons are trying to say...

Even now, it is difficult to see.
Even now, it is difficult to be.

Even right now, it is **finding** its way out.
Even right now, it is finding its way in.

A silent transition,
an unseen broken connection,

a **frozen** fish.

My broken neurons are trying to say
that it is OK to be lost.

My broken neurons are trying to say that it is OK to ask for **help**.

My broken neurons are trying to say:
"My darling, stay alive".

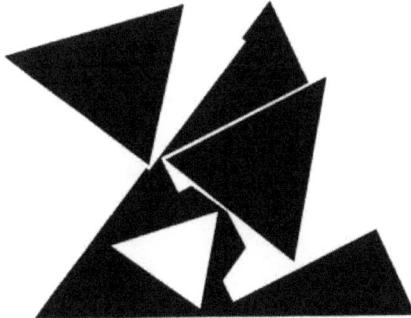

Spoon_07 : Psalms in my Palms

Uncertain times of re-lived trauma
too much for my heart today,
too much for my mind to take this time.

I break at the point of melting down,
with strong currents of tear tides,
it was not my intention to lose my shine.

In this mountain of deep suffering,
I have found a light in blue,
and I am now aware of the existence

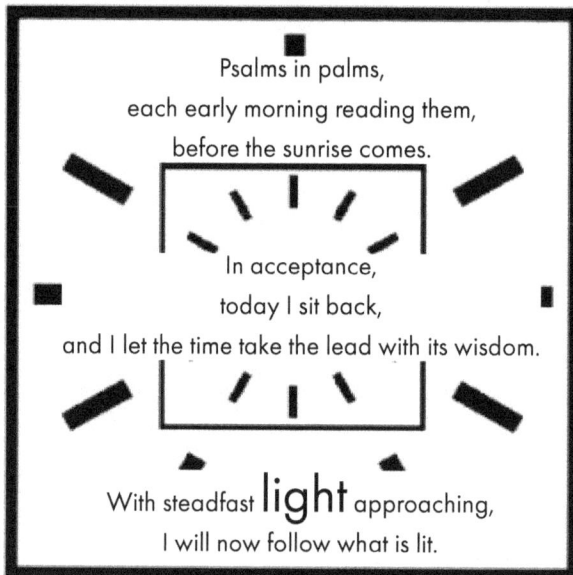

of your unique you.

Psalms in palms,
each early morning reading them,
before the sunrise comes.

In acceptance,
today I sit back,
and I let the time take the lead with its wisdom.

With steadfast light approaching,
I will now follow what is lit.

Spoon_08 : I Praise You

Dear mother-father God,
help me see the blue in this
and direct me to the timely answer.

Breathe in – breathe out.
Breathe out – breathe in.

"Where did you come from?" - the moon asks.
I try to joke in my answer,
but I know where I come from...
...and it's not fun.

I come from deep pain.
I come from being a broken hourglass...
with the glass and thinnest sand now gone.

I come from forgetting how to walk,
and had to learn again.
Step-by-step,
with my bare feet on uneven grounds.

But it does not matter where I come from.

It matters that I am here now.

And that I am here with you.
I know at times I lose my spirit
I know at times I make you sad, but please forgive me.

I praise you.

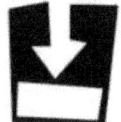

Spoon_09 : Powerlessly Empowered

As a **breaking** lightning in the sky I start to crack my jelly brain.

Rationally trying to control the force,
...here I am completely powerless.

Powerless
in face of such a beautiful blue color
that brings me back to that sky.

Powerless
as a light feather
that safely flies supported by a gentle breeze.

Powerless
to life dynamics that are bigger than us
and that shows us our path.

Powerless

in being **pulled** by this light
which then energizes my soul and heart.

And with the **energy** given to me
I get empowered.

Powerlessly empowered by you.

Spoon_10 : Simple is good for me today

Simple is good for me today.

As the sunrise catches my eyes

I can now swim to the buoy.

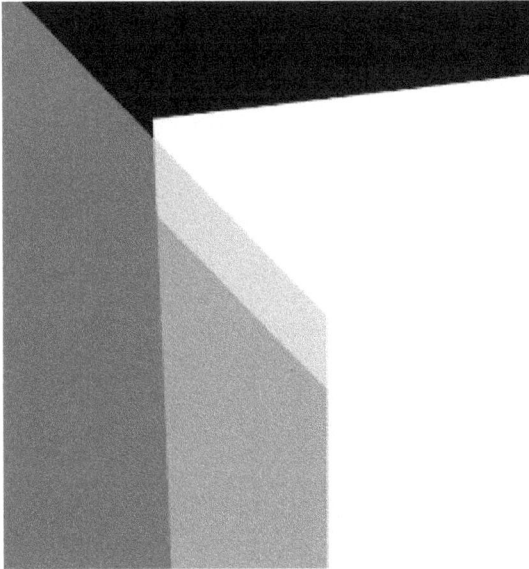

As I walk up the hill, I can feel my legs crying out.

As I put the butter on my toast

I see your **smile** in my head.

As I do nothing much
I can still dream today.

Simple is very very good for me today.

Spoon_11 : To Peaceful Madness

I look 4 peace.
I look 4 calm.

I look into rationalizing the self and the surrounding as a process of letting go. In search of peace and calm madness, which I think we all have in some respect in our variable

patterns of textured light.

I spend the days looking at analyzing painted details and also bigger pictures, shaping thoughts into reflective matter.

As I value and need that extra light in pragmatism and self-reflection I also want to internalize the positivity of the real emotional madness of my soul. Sea-ing things differently does not hurt. It empowers my feelings. Feelings that can then direct me into allowing an emotionally driven pilot of greater intelligence. Something of a greater current, something of a greater hug, something of a greater us.

Driving the self in the chaotic surrounding, patterns are starting to form in an automatic

move through the **storm**. Storm of emotional discoveries, allowing the right

exploration of inner existence as well as outer **being**.

Looking for that greater power outside the self, maybe escaping the reality of my limits, or maybe just embracing them. Solitude is a space of peaceful strength in fragility, searching for answers of patterns and tempos, like a particle that is floating (and yet firmly standing) in the unknown.

So, maybe, renewing the self in a peaceful madness; a madness of accepting that the answer does not always come from me,
and neither does the question.

Spoon_12 : In Millions of Slow Beats

In millions of slow beats
my five senses are cracking in motion of unrest.

In millions of slow beats,
my mind travels at high speed.

In millions of slow beats,

my heart responds to the walk.

In millions of slow beats,

I can see that great sight.

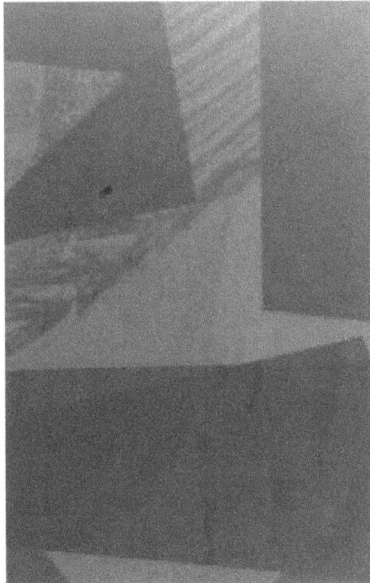

Spoon_13 : I'd Gladly Fly

I'd gladly fly
to that island I was born in.
Tomorrow, today, now.

I'd gladly fly
if I didn't have these broken wings.

I am trying to rehabilitate them,

but I cannot **control** them as I used to.

Sometimes I manage to fly a little,
even for a while longer than yesterday,
but I then recognize that pattern of pain,
of dizziness,
of cognitive dangerous illusion and
I just have to try to land
as safe as I can.

And **the**n...in vertigo,
I cannot move.
And then...
I actually would have preferred to have crash-landed.

And then...
I actually don't want to be anymore.

But then the **wind** picks me up,
and shows me the way of being again.

And so, I start again,
and I can say that I'd gladly fly again.

Spoon_14 : To the Higher Presence Care

Using rationale to help shape sight, embracing into a direction of luminous sensation which is hard not to see now, never mind not to follow. In steps of thoughtfulness, and leaving deep traces, the pathway appears a bit unsteady in its essence of perception.
It kinda varies in its needed gear.
Not that I think that everything needs to be set in gear properly, but it would be nice to have a bit of help in the climbing of this hill, especially when everything else in life is in a constant climbing action.

Could you please give me an indication for a more steady moving forward? Could you please turn, just at points the hill upside down? Could you please give me a gentle push towards that gorgeous blue?

I know that I must find the right place by myself. And I think I have actually found it in my heart. And those torments of closure experience and inability of being who I was, they are now softly landing down.
Landscapes of gardens, some in need of watering, some in need of pruning.
Show me the way, I embrace your presence, and I will walk with you and blue.

"Dear Mother-Father God, give us the strength of stepping forward in gentle jumps.

With a clear feeling of respectful processes that keeps my life in your hands, and our hearts in your heart.

I am dizzy today from vertigo spells, and my mind is hurting me like never before, and my heart is not feeling well either now. Please give us a sign. Be with us in our journey of finding blue peace, and in all the moments that this will require and that you have already lined up for us. I am suffering in invisible pain, and I need a bit of stability to reframe and reshape, with this blue angel of my soul.

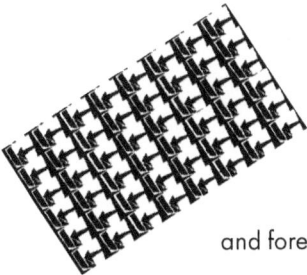

Dear Mother-Father God,
I know you will take us forever with you

and forever we trust your immense deep blue."

Spoon_15 : Nature Designs Me

Nature designs me
in river flowing

of a **rumbling** stream.

Shadows of clouds
passing by as I fall

down

the tallest tree.

Oh, seven birds flying through
Oh, three squirrels jumping out
Oh, twenty-two salmon swimming up.

Nature designs us
in patterns that we cannot control
in those vibrant seeds of existence.

Design the next phase of life
shaping holes into the abyss

drawing **segments** of dropping tears.

Nature designs everything
as I take the next road
and as I stop to close the bike chain
once and for all.

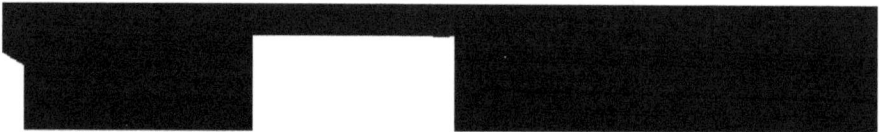

Spoon_16 : In Cage

When I opened that box
I did not know what to expect.

Certainly not what I have found
and certainly not such a **weird** smell.

A little bird
with dirty wings
in a dirty rusty cage.

Dead. Stuffed. Taxidermied as it looks.

In that moment I moved forward
and in a twist of **spiral** turns
I ended up in the cage myself.

I was inside the dirty mess
I was inside that dirty bird
I was attached to those dirty **wings!**

Oh my goodness me
I am that bird I first saw.

Am I dead?
Am I stuffed?
Am I taxidermied as I look?

So I seem to.

But you can be certain
that I will soon start to move again.

Spoon_17 : Glossy Insomnia

The elevator opens.
Am I on another equally important beat?
Indistinct ringing.

A whole kit of lavender
to keep the lights on
under the pillow of that bed.

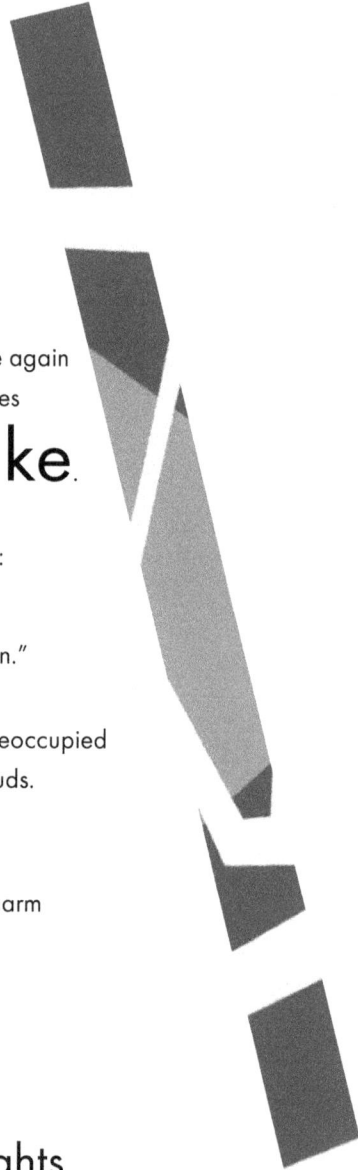

Becoming someone people can see again
with dark circles around my eyes

frankly pretending I am **awake**.

Diamond as a clear message:
"Take your best shot
as you might not f**in**d me again."

Only two hundred times I have been preoccupied
of being a survivor of public clouds.

A woman's bible to discover
with the intention of not causing harm
but going deeper into belief.

Thank you for that,
for staying awake with me
in those long and **golden nights**.

Spoon_18 : A broken record

This is it.

This is the **beginning**.

I don't like you much.

I think I'm paranoid
in popular smart cool
of exceptional shitty pedigree.

It turns.

"Oh ... don't worry, I got you!"

It turns.

"Oh ... it's a **last** ditch effort".

It turns.

"Oh ... I don't have to defend myself".

A broken record of globally final stages
as an **opportunity** to a fresh start
dancing in purple lights.

Move your legs!
Relax in laughter.
Advance into the infinite corridor
of darkness at night.

Spoon_19 : Hospital Night

A **little** big but they are clean,
and I am walking in them
as I now want to scream.

Safety and comfort my ass...
...they are not my goal now
as I just wanna fight
in this limbo of weird nonsense.

Misunderstanding the minute of negligence?
Miscommunicating the freak out in cleaner sheets?
Oh dear, where is the registry?

"Oh f*ck"...sorry..."Oh dear"
it's been a long week
of groans and sighs and **worries**.

Exhaling, chuckling, kissing.

Breathing a plastic smell
of apparent cleaned rooms in antibacterial spray
and everything feels so cold.

Thanks for taking me here...
...thanks for leaving me here...
...thanks as always for believing in me.

Currently in low risk
of harming self
and harming others.

Currently an image of **trees**

hanging in the thoughts but with no current intent.

Depressive disorder jumping up, depressive disorder digging in.

Planned attempt of switching **of**f,
in overload and swimming out,
currents of being alive.

Capable in appearance and behavior, sorting through waves of medication,
daily bringing in the focus.

Rehabilitation interventions not complete

but increasing hopes in **circumstance**
of life changes of disability.

It appears anywhere, suddenly turning dark and quickly defying progression.

Low risk becomes high risk so quickly.
And now what?

Spoon_21 : Pressing

Deterioration in **mental** health pressing who we are.
Inability of thinking straight.
Symptomatology of depressive patterns.

Psychiatrist intervention in balance of behaviors,
continuing management of reconfigured self.

Increasing further cycle of such emotions
that bring us down in a few minutes
and build up in manic symptoms.

Running impact of neuro physio
shaping into artistic healthier means
that only you can **read** into.

Consultations of clinical specialists
often floating in noisy activity

of pills and drug **intake** and more.

Pressing down the belly button.
Pressing up behind the ear.
Pressing in the middle broken field.

At one stage expressing pain,
at one stage necessitating changes,
all is lost in the wilderness of the mind.

Spoon_22 : I am trying

I had a choice to make that day.
Do something different.
Do something **kind**.

Confusing time in spelling phrases
of **tasteless** pains
in chronic begging of a new chance.

Stop with the self pitying bullshit,
stand now into new vocabulary,
in pensive music all around.

Indistinct slam of emotions,
in upper level of a building pillow
with shiny windows reflecting in my eyes.

I say that I can make it.
Orchestral love takes me up,
in seconds I am flying to catch the star.

Flowers of fading times,
I always thought to be within,
and yet I am here today in this new **place**.

I am trying. I am trying.
I really am trying.

Spoon_23 : Chocolate

Dark.

Moonlight through the window
with tiny Iggy under blanket
and with the clock ticking by.

An attempt to make me smile,
a reflection of a lighting in the **sky**
all brought forward into the cliff.

The pier of black silhouettes
moving left and right
at the sound of the floating band.

The storm is very close.
My tea is cooling off.
And the horizon is not in line.

In smoothness feel of constant now,
with sweet taste of **bitter** being,
I now move forward.

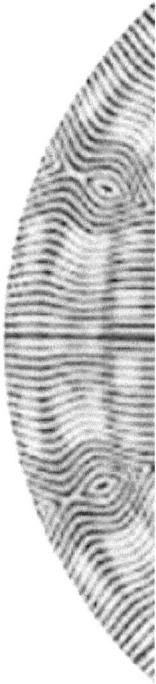

Spoon_24 : Even Longer

Like that feel in your eyes
when you are slowly getting up
having a longer morning drink.

Almost like an invisible quiet weight
that call for closing shops
and put your back at rest.

Even longer than a moment.
Even longer than a **dream**.
Even longer than you thought it would be.

Blanket of soft wool
with calming waves in the disc
with sunny spectrums of glass **and** skin.

Little birds of **nourish**ed sunrise, walking down the beach
and floating in the sea.

Take off your clothes.
Jump in water. Stay still.

Even longer than a moment.
Even longer than a dream.
Even longer than you thought it would be.

Spoon_25 : When we fall asleep.

We were waiting over there.
Water coming down the roofs.
Is it too late?

An orange tree
immediately losing fruit as I pass by,
absence of decisions in your mind.

A statement, stubborn as I was.
A change in your voice
sliding the door of angel words.

I wanted it so badly,
to understand, to listen to those needs
in the name of poor me as stupid as I am.

A boat **of** troubles and questions,
devastated you and me,
investigating who we were.

When we fall asleep we recognize the feel,
a simple gentle **hug** in touching bodies
that has silently waited to speak again.

When we fall asleep I'm convinced you can hear me,
desperate to find a way for us,
desperate to lose paranoia: "I love you".

Spoon_26 : Bells of Water

Lacked in good motivation,
arguing under column of curly olive trees
whilst following a morning of constant questions.

Without a warning of defense,
getting closer to vitally important feel
of testimony from another world.

Moving backwards in blue tragedy
of riding horses within trees,
I jump into a deep black hole.

Dazzling reliable judgments
walking down the corridors
with no lights around me.

A silver lining of a special moment,
wearing a seatbelt whilst standing still,
on a wooden boat full of water.

Ringing bells getting over us,
covering our whispers of hope
for that end to come.

Spoon_27 : Mirror

Worried about health and future,
looking into my reflected mirrored eyes
in a long road of chestnut trees.

Door to door, calling loneliness
as a guardian of a diagnosis
that has left me here and there.

You always leave the window open,
this is us, convincing ourselves
of options entangled in the rope.

Do you remember it?
For a **long** time I looked at you
in the mirror of parallel limits.

I was looking for my previous self
that is now **gone** into the abyss
of broken neurons there to speak.

I am nobody here.
Inside here, an empty soul,
perhaps with a **possibility** of redemption.

Spoon_28 : Hot Milk

In deep night darkness I am awake,
overloaded by a day of stimuli
that has built up into much pain.

In dizzy waves I try to close my eyes,
and in silent matter I create
atmosphere of calming rooms.

Boiling milk on the stove
and turning in a wheat cocoa
for another woken night.

With autumnal vibes of fresh air
I sit in the corner of the patio
lighting a sweet orange candle.

Sipping hot milk from the uneven mug,
I put the tiles together
of that unbalanced wall of cards.

Burning curtains of waxed textiles,
I might find a bit of warmth,
I might find a bit of love.

Only two left, and it's just 11am.
It has been a little too much already
just walking down to the beach.

Surrounded by painful everyday sounds

the energy is hitting **blank**

and I need to get the **extra** spoons.

Only one left, and it's just 1pm.
I need to rest, I need to balance today better,
I need to keep a little more for later.

Nothing left, and it's just 5pm.
I am done for the day.

More pills.
Time to let go.
Bed.

Sleep.

See you tomorrow.

Cutting through the pain
burning surface skin
forgetting what it is.

Waking up with injured face
no idea what happened there
only feeling upside down.

It happens like a swift rush of sun
but it's a deep burnt of segments
becoming scars on trapped skin.

Sitting down in that white noise
trying to memorize the action
that detachment has now gone.

Wondering man walking lovely
thinking math of self awareness
crying of yet loosen memories.

I feel out of my persona, not recording simple gestures, not recording scattered slaps.

I am not sure what to do
in psychotic heavy episodes
to immaterial salty death.

Spoon_31 : Waking Up to singing Wren

Waking up to singing wren
it's a dream I can now live
with this genuine gifted being.

Stepping up to new directions
slowly finding deeper spoons,
now engaging in parent_hood.

Breaking down with little squirrel,
fighting back to stand again
and climbing in orchards for that apple.

Messy matters are now the norm,
untidy spaces of loving sweetness
never ending where you guessed.

Waking up to singing wren,
it's as like I never knew
that loving tenderness could be.

Looking up to the sky,
silhouettes of long thin branches
are appearing in the view.

Little squirrel is jumping off,
with open wings of wren sweet thing,
now moving gently in the air.

Have a good flight my squirrel-wren.

Spoon_32 : I can't afford

I can't afford disorder,
I've got too much inside.

I can't afford disorder,
I've read it too many times.

I can't afford disorder,
please call it condition.

I can't afford disorder,
my brain can get quite lost.

I can't afford disorder,
it can be dangerous for me.

I can't afford disorder,
in each moment of my day.

I can't afford disorder,
as my spoon will empty soon.

I just can't afford it,
and I am tired of explaining.

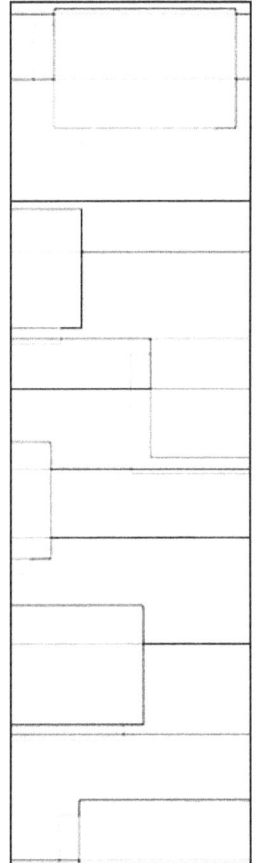

Spoon_33 : I don't want to let go

My head feels like an exploding balloon,
chronic migraine of intense light,
with a sounding pitch over the moon.

I hate all of this.
I hate all of me.
I want to die.

Daily pills taken away from me,
as in danger of let go,

and so I am fed like I'm mad.

I don't know what else to do.
Quiet please. That's only what I ask.
Quiet, please. I beg you all.

I don't want to let go.
I have already lost a deep part of me,
I don't want to lose another one.

My tiny Tootsie sits next to me.
She is so tender and strong for me.
She doesn't even realize how huge she is.

I am feeling like I cannot move.
I am feeling like this isn't me.
I am feeling like I should let go.

But writing this makes me shake.
And ask for help as I can.

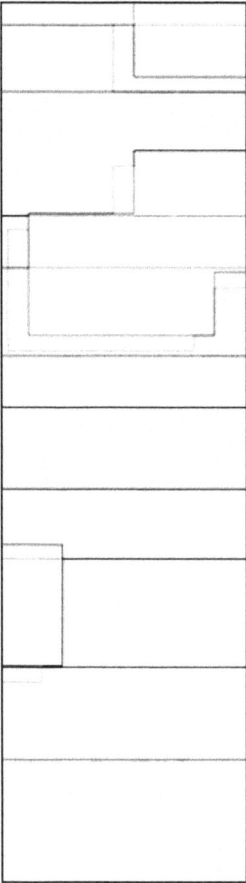

Spoon_34 : I am sorry for the language.

I am sorry for the language.
But that f**king med is f**ing f**k.
I don't just like to use bad words,

but trust me that you would have also had enough.

Anti-psychotic as my friends?
"They help you...they are there to make you feel better, to function."

Oh, really...and why I am sO f**king out now?

Why do I need these meds to drive me more crazy?
Right now...not sure what the f**k is happening,

but it is losing me in f**king f**k.

I am sorry for the language.
I really am.
This isn't me.

Spoon_35 : Find a way

Could I stay here by myself?

Currently unavailable,
with ringing eyes telling me
that I need to sleep.

Why?
Because it means something to me.

Nearly everything.
And I think you can see that too.

How do we open the gate?
Is there a code I cannot find?
Is there a way to trespass?

#whatever

I need to open that gate.
I need to find a **way**.

Spoon_36 : Friends of Walk

An imaginary place of crystal water
reflecting singing women of sunny light,
white and blue in longer vowels.

A photo. An image of long windows,
with falling leaves flowing inside,
o'clock - it's dinner time!

Should we bring some elaborate concept,
an **organized mess** of mathematician mind,
with our thick glasses as magnetic opposites?

Crying child in the buggy, moving forward,
dirty goofy view **of** astigmatism,
trying to make a picture.

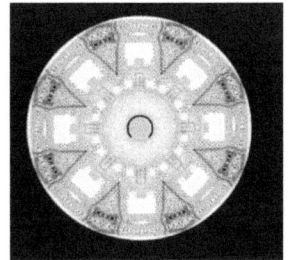

Sitting uncomfortably in extension
we listen to the birds on the acer,
we listen to nothing else left behind.

Friends of walk,
waiting in customized settings,
deep down in a program of **audacity**.

Tomorrow, we will assess regulations,
experimenting on assumptions
of that tall infinite wall.

Spoon_37 : People to talk to...

Mournful ideas of transmitting sadness,
with sighs of self-burning
to disguise the pain.

Sit now. I cannot bear it.
I have been put in harm and it hurts.
Is this **meaningful** for something?

I have to be strong.
We have to be.

Positive and accepting.

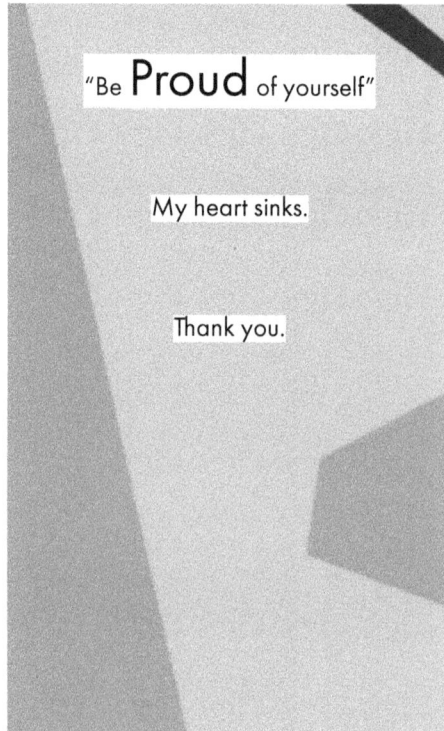

"Be **Proud** of yourself"

My heart sinks.

Thank you.

Retrieve your items and go.
Toying with your scraping eyes,
I washed into the sink.

I can't be here.
Neither there...
...nor over-there.

It's like escaping realities
into dissociated thoughts of movement
that makes no sense of being.

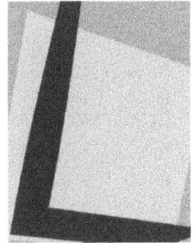

Maybe I forget that there might be a reason.
Maybe.
Maybe.

Was it a coincidence?
Was it needed to find the way?
Keep your distance.

Empty cupboards of rotten dreams,
toasting fire of damned grenades
created by hallucinations without meaning.

Inspecting shelves of opaque glass,
whilst a toilet smell of boiled
conserved frogs.

Spoon_39 : Nothingness

Residing under a mattress
it's my notebook
depicting waves and rolls of late **nights**.

Everything walks around a grieving time.
Everything can look out for you now.
Everything convinces me that it will be OK.

Yellow strings of silhouettes
standing in the middle of the field
with crows picking their heads off.

Transparent boxes full of leaves,
sculpting seafront of gray clouds
into corridors **of naked trees**.

Borders of nothing
yet to be released
into a peace agreement.

Neurons fighting in cool spirit,
needing rounds of wild garlic
and growing spicy in the guts.

Alcohol-free
painted into pages
of nothingness.

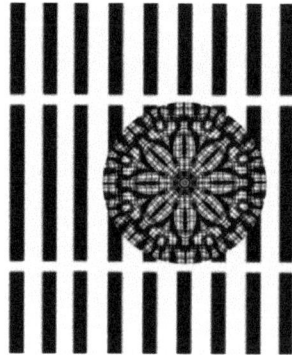

Spoon_40 : A race of Smiles

Sorry it's late,
but I was lost in the forest
with no sign of a way out.

Tall trees with complex branches
of metal structures
in the air.

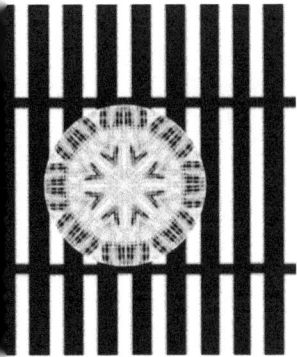

A robot bird nesting gold,
tweets a hurricane
out of beak.

What would happen?
Recognising shaving heads
in the overgrown hedge.

What a mess of gestures,
in blocks of fighting spirits
with PVC in their biodiverse skins.

Clear sky,
intelligent processor of plasters
and daily pills.

A race of smiles stays with me.
A race of tears flows away.

Spoon_41 : As We Speak

Forgiveness is the highest form of love.
Anonymous love of splendid green grass in October rain,
pouring down like frozen matters from nowhere.

Church bells in the distance
with gremlins jumping up and down
as the rhythm grows in speedy allegro.

Labradors, Spaniels and Greyhounds
running free at low tide lowest,
what a race to have.

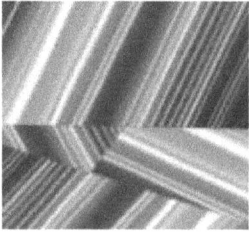

Cold dips in the ocean as it is,
freezing essence of mind and body
warming later in cups of tea.

Sunlight shining, what a gift
as the seafront stroll of longest way
turns into fermenting flowers of crab-apples.

On a bench I have refuge
with light fresh breeze on my face
and a bandage on my broken eyebrow.

Kissing sun of dreamy day,
I am waiting for sweet blue squirrel,
here and then
as we speak.

Spoon_42 : Something Great

Can we talk about this?
In framed pictures of our **memories**,
I see the love we had in us.

Invisible silent steps
knitting blinds of mashed thoughts
under a rain jacket of blue leather.

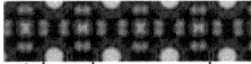

A last dance together
in a turbine of succulent plants
with pink flowers turning out.

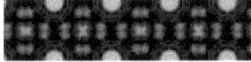

It's clouding up,
needing assistance in circles
as central streets in western town.

Yellow line of traditions
instructing us of basic lectures,
I ain't no-one's "Bitch"!

For the rest of that signed agreement,
I am here to stay
and wait for **you**.

Chatters of something great.
Chatters of something friendly.
Chatters of furious hope.

Spoon_43 : H2O

As a beetle living in plain wooden house,
existing in dropping drops,
I am glad to be here today.

Ice-cream van cycling across,
strawberry vanilla cone
with choco tears at your **choice**.

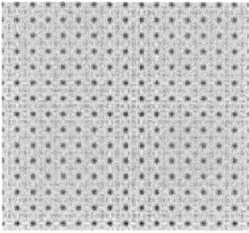

Do you remember that?
Could you have guessed?

Things are going to be easier,
fading screen of welcome news,
brain catching up for a double flip.

There I am, in the air,
I see myself falling down,

I see myself diving **in**.

Reflective tiles of coloured glass
all in line,
all in order.

In blue water I am now moving,
touching depth of H^2O
and staying deep down with my soul.

Spoon_44 : Unwrapping Photos

Overcome my anger,
overcome my fear,
overcome my own self.

Pink bougainvillea
creeping strongly on the house
and hugging it softly with its spiky branches.

Light music that secretly sits there,
hanging on to the moment we kissed
unwrapping photos of our memories.

Train stations passing by,
framed by metal windows
speeding into tunnels of white lights.

Ten to nine anxious at arrival,
busy central square of **madness**,
guaranteed vertigo spin.

I tried not to lose the road,
with the map of nonsense lines,
unsuitable for reception of directions.

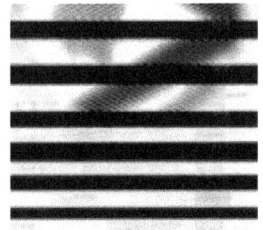

Capital mistakes that I still want to make,
bringing drawings of a **tomorrow**
I will turn around to a new day.

Spoon_45 : To a Lighter Tomorrow

One more time,
slow imperfections of tenderness,
I miss you dearest friend.

A bundle of nervous nerves
taking a wrong decision
that changed things forever then.

Cabins on white rocks,
structured in wood,
you certainly know that engineering.

Permaculture in surrounding lands,
with self-grown ideas
of seeded times.

Under a bush I lay still,
cuddling bones of crystal paper
that draw butterflies on woolen flowers.

Missing the turning pages of a script,
now lost on Netflix longer list.

Spotlights of triangles and lines,
in breaking leaves of daily matters,
seasons move to a lighter tomorrow of nowhere.

Spoon_46 : Heaters Off

Stepping away from there,
awake in starry sky
I stand with swans around the lake.

Details of staring **eyes**,
enclosing songs of homeland
attached in strings of cotton.

Moving through the tears,
in music **never** recorded
curled up in my pajamas.

Placing nightmares in the mirror,
categorized in boxes never opened
now buried in the woods.

Heaters off,
convincing my guts of what is there,
warming up in understanding clauses.

Slow mental spirits of solutions
haunted in controlled acts
missing docks of South-East London.

Shots of vodka laughing non-sense,
feeling really **shuttered** now,
time to catch a cab to avoid the rain.

Spoon_47 : Remembrance

Accidental hit of extreme strength,
shocked in warning of danger,
as the jump that still haunts me.

A message of throwing witches,
turning off the picked martyr,
rebooting as a young lad's life.

Architecture of green squared units,
far **back** re-envisioned
and only now reconstructed.

Images of us running under thunders
crossing bridges of resolutions
under a twisted lamp-post with no lights.

Cleaning mochas of espressos,
parked in the middle of the green
with pink-blue pears in the basket.

Gentle shower of **brandy** drinks
in tough evenings with gins of awaken mind
hugged in **sex** as floating bodies.

Jogging nights of shrunk cold heads
wearing hats of sailors' travels,
opening ears for remembrance.

It

will

never

bloody

work,

with

so

so...

...so so,

so so...

...NOThing.

Spoon_49 : Caught between the Fences

I was gone early,
exhaling indistinct whispers
always counting my own fingers.

Sitting in the idle of the woods,
with **racing** mind I need to slow
for dreams to shape another door.

Cheers to day by day,
tasting **spicy** on my lips
and turning sweet within my tears.

Panting glorious sex
opening heavy stuck doors
in understanding **jaguar** skins.

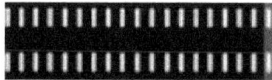

A smile that breaks the self
down below terrified
like no one else here to come.

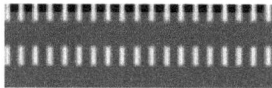

Destiny of our choices,
burning in sharp thin bites
caught between the fences.

Coloured glass and buzzing walks,
a little too much out of it
embracing me for the rest of days.

Spoon_50 : I do love to dance.

I do love to dance.
Shame I spin in seconds
of me trying a nice new move.

Oh, I do love to dance.
Shame I cannot listen to music
no matter what.

Oh, I do love to dance.
And so in memories I do,
didn't we have such good fun?

But hey, I do love to dance.
Now, under raining sounds
of gentle stormy weather.

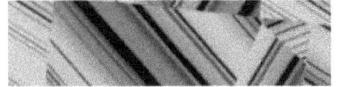

Yes, I do love to dance.
And closing my eyes sitting still in the field,
I move following winds and leaves.

I absolutely love to dance.
Just, who would have thoughts
in how many different ways.

I do love to dance.
But I really really miss
dancing with you.

Spoon_51 : In binary terms.

In binary terms of zeros and ones,
the code disrupts the social platform
of who we were and who we are.

Reloading tags of pictured selves,
in blocking options from the user
I now want to program more.

Interfaces of coded lights
in gram of **instant** feel
followed by the unknown.

Liking hearts of simple message
neither writing a few words
neither putting any thoughts.

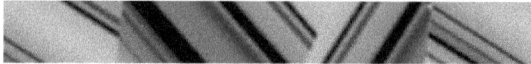

Refresh the page of multi-content
in **line** with square type cluster B,
personality recording from the cam.

Whatsapping loving thoughts,
in corners of misreadings,
there it builds for thirty minutes.

Time **to shut down** now.

Time to power off.

Spoon_52 : Invis_Ability

It is difficult to see inside my head.

I try to look **behind** my eyes...
I try to look inside the ears...
...and through the nose...
...and in the mouth...

...but still I cannot see what is inside **my** head.
At times I really would like to see what is inside...
...especially when I have a massive headache

or when I see that all is foggy
or when I get my fainty moments.
I really would like to see what is inside...
...especially when I hear those painful sounds

or when my head does crazy **spins**
or when that ringing never stops.

I really would like to see what is inside...

...especially when I only see those white lights

or when I forget what I am just doing
or when I can only lay in bed.

But it is so difficult to see inside my head

and sometimes I get so upset because I cannot understand.

It is difficult to see inside my head for me but also for everyone else

...and so I have to write it down: Not All Disabilities are Visible!

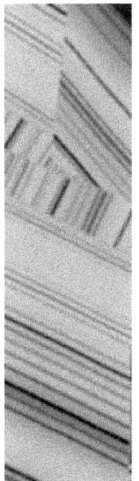

Spoon_53 : Random Dream

At a wedding with Dudessa,

not sure where this is
I **turn** around
and so much noise.

In a moment we are running through the corridor
which then becomes a tiny stream
opening up into a lake.

Hold on ... it was a lake,
now we are swimming from Sardinia,
popping up in Si-ci-ly,
final stop in gentle Greece.

Oh, hold on again.
We are in a woodland,
no way I have a rifle in my hands,
hunting wild boars in my flip-flops turned boots?

Wake **up** Luca.
No idea what that all means.

Time for coffee **now**.

Maybe message Dudessa.

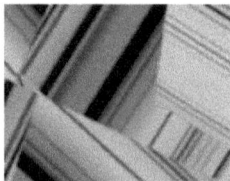

Spoon_54 : In Mental of Me Brain

In mental illness of me brain
I write lines of nothingness
as I feel **naked** on open day.

Nothingness shaping something
and so materializing thoughts
into possible analysis of **self**.

At times it is very dark.
At times it is very painful.
At times it does not flow.
At times I just let go.

In verses of ink in paper
anywhere I could write down
it gives freedom to me brain.

I thank poetry for allowing me to be,
with heavy matters that come afloat
and now we go for a long **swim**.

A combination of emotions
that might not usually reflect the feel,
in rhythm space of lines and commas.

Limited in any manner,
I stand and try.

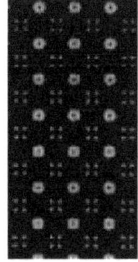

Spoon_55 : To New Green Shoots

Tattoos of something to remember,
as identity shifts in burnt agenda
and the mark will stay forever.

Piercing writing on the skin:
I am following the line,
I am following the ink.

Painful neck of standing still:
martyr pattern of cracking jokes,
shaving heads in a metal patch.

Antennas disconnected from the hand
external only to themselves
giving signals of false direction.

Let's make peace in this gray morning,
let's forget the dried leaves of anger
and move on to new green shoots.

Spoon_56 : Surfing a Wave of Peaceful Clouds

Surfing **a** wave of peaceful clouds
in a **tunnel** without end
I move curling up on my knees.

Shadow under water follows me in each turn, I am now scared to fall down.

Gripping strongly on the board
I turned the other way
but the cylinder is closing off on me.

I turn again towards the light but never ending in the way,
the shadows are getting much closer now.

Naked bodies sitting near the shore
on a spiky bench of bougainvillea
tied into a bamboo grid.

Camomile flowers
flowering into my glass of vodka straight,
adjusted to sweet bitter lime.

Rings around the body structure
posing risk of no return,
I drink to all that is to happen.

Hong-Kong mugs of indo-spresso
with no sugar left behind
and with milk drips that are out-dated.

The tunnel turns into a sphere
with no exit
and no secret ways.

Spoon_57 : Anti Nothing

Previous letters unresponded;
in signature they failed me,
turning pointed forks into a date.

Prunes with no stones left inside
going down with the pills

or Sertra **swings** and quiet **pins**.

Anti nothing I dissolve
and ask you whether this is it?,
as a line not to cross.

Little squirrel **jumps** in front
clearly making a good sign
clearly saying "Baba, just stand-by".

I love you dearly my sweet blue,
in all your tones kept in you,
I'll try my best, I swear, I'll do.

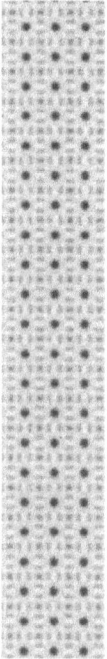

You

Lose

a

Sock

in

every

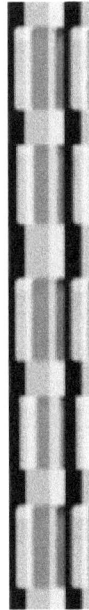

Wash.

Spoon_59 : Fluo Pedals

Rowing the boat with rolling eyes
I stir here and there
to avoid the current.

Not sure if I am able to anchor down,
working support of clear needs,
trying to write it in acceptance.

I move from A to B,
in **muddy** land of soaking boots,
with awesome flowers popping up
as rain and sun fight their way.

Set-up a **bloody** taxi account,
buying that bike with 30 electrics,
opening heart for fluorescent pedals.

Draw a line of possibility,
on seaside seafront **flow**,
cycling ways of balance strength.

In stillness I am moving.

Spoon_60 : Salvation of Liberation

News moves around
of the birth of
u-ni-ty.

Expeditions are organized to mark the day forever,
with kings and queens
following stars
but getting lost in
thunder-storm.

Progressive and alternative ways of finding paths,
kings of mountains and queens of rivers,
land on lakes of
juicy **pears**.

Animals meeting up and sharing fruits,
the news keeps **traveling**
and reach new kingdoms,
in water,
air
and
mother earth.

U-Ni-Ty
is all we have
for a peaceful life we all deserve.

Spoon_61 : In Times of Lost Spirit

In times of lost spirit
we travel far to find the source.

Finding patterns
and mapping explanations,
we sail in the air
to find the route.

A route that yet it is to shape,
a route that yet it is to be,
a route that yet it is to crack.

Rivers, seas, lands
of **parallel** ventures,
we flow in **currents**
to a sudden deja-vu.

Spoon_62 : In Seasons of Virginian Creeping Brain

CNS autumnal functioning
in neuro creeping of Virginia
impaired as the seasons change.

Reflections in tender rain,
forgetting empty matters
of invisible neu-ron-s.

Organic evolution of Sun creations
moving up through the patio,
and shifting pastels in cold pantone.

Regaining warmer balance
in mental health of broken ladder,
as Nature does it best.

A labyrinth of hedged paths
covering journeys of nothingness
now coloring the pain.

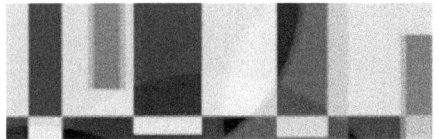

Can **YOU** imagine
not listening to it?

Can you imagine
just leaving it behind?

Can you imagine
all the people,
and so many people?

Imagine

Gone.

Spoon_64 : Bobbin' on

Solar panels in the eyes,
sunbathing looking up,
waves breaking on.

Warming hearts of silent creatures,
bobbin' on
a floating board.

Seagulls looking for break-fast
children chatting their way out
detectors beeping metal nothing.

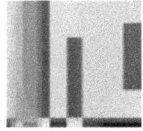

Attention, "Oh, Cocco Bello!",
wanna single or double cone?

Ocean freezing simple thoughts
triangles sailing higher tide
no-one waiting on the side.

Wheeling tat of toos
on me arms and on me leg,
now we are going back to back.

Spoon_65 : Guess What?

Something more neutral.
Are you mad at me?
Wonderful.

Fusing yes and nos,
I turn around
backing up a straight maybe.

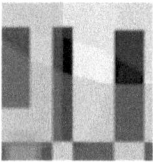

Photos, photos, photos.
Guess what?
Unfocused.

Spotlight of qualified headache
with nice haircut crazy lines,
they are the ones completely mad.

A ghost with deep unsettling feel
lost in the romance of desire,
strangely wanting another chance.

Step by step in arguing dreams,
healthy in psycho anal-ysis
in a waste of a thousand beats.

Spoon_66 : As a Shutter of the Sun

Dry soil in a container
what a
scene.

Two yellow flowers as a shutter
of the
Sun.

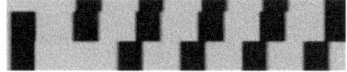

One bloody snail bites the leaf,
WT
F!

Tall the stems are coming
out of the
pack.

Oh my,
Oh my,
Oh my.

Both flowers are now clearly touched.

Spoon_67 : Centers of Outskirt Being

Outskirts of centered beings
flowing in blue bells
of trust wood - land.

Sudden **spell** of light
reaches mountains of desire,
and
outskirts of centered beings
appear on the silent map.

A journey of discovery
that not only breaks the border
but also cracks the epicenter.

Neurons travel at light speed
left to right,
up
and
down.

Shadows **of linear** obstacles
appear in mental steadiness,
keeping moving as a circle
nothing changes
and
nothing happens.

In centers of outskirt being
we find a new way.

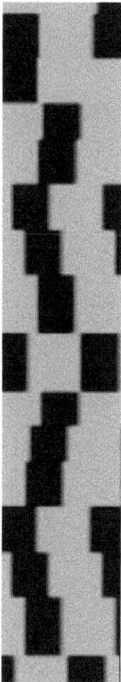

The brain is such a **complex** thing.

Floating
particles
move
around.

Self linking
creates
what
we think.

Connections
change
in many
ways.

Neuroscience
opening to what
is not

the **norm**.

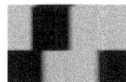

No brain is the same.

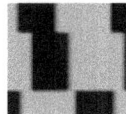

Spoon_69 : Wren Wren Wran

Wren-egading in the park
in quick jumps here and there
little Squirrel is singing songs:

Wren Wren Wran
Wron Wren Wrun
Wrin Wron Wren!

Wren-lentless flying around
making spins of spinning ways
he moves swiftly in disguise.

Sailing boats of inter-im
following eagles in the sky
singing songs of twitter-ing:

Wren Wren Wran
Wron Wren Wrun
Wrin Wron Wren!

Then I wake up; it's just a dream.
I walk down the stairs and all is quiet.
Nothing there.
So I sit and
whisper in missing Squirrel:

Wren Wren Wran
Wron Wren Wrun
Wrin Wron Wren.

Celebrating a request
for reading **more**.

Sending right file
and no **track** changes.

Timeline saying
it's been a month.

Patience is what I need.

I am scared and yet excited.

Pinging email of double 0.

It's a no.

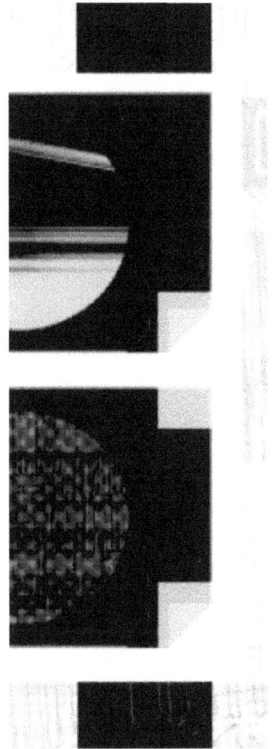

Morning Glory of the abyss,
can I ask you a question?

Sure, go ahead.

What are you waiting for?

I am not waiting.
I am just pondering
what
the
right
decision
might
be.

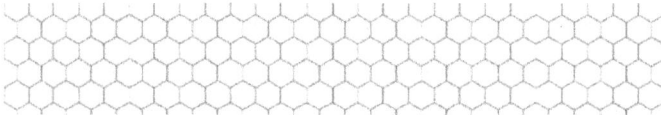

A kiss to the way we are,

an arrow for direction.

A kiss to hope,

an arrow for standing up.

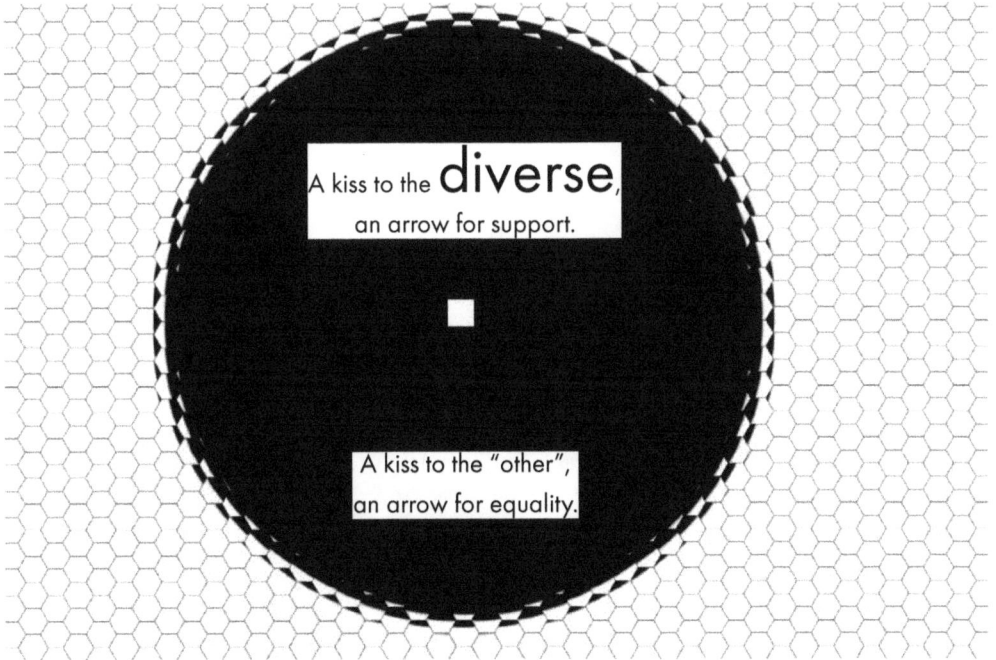

A kiss to the diverse,
an arrow for support.

A kiss to the "other",
an arrow for equality.

Spoon_73 : Eco Car

The eco car sits near the pavement.
No sign of **moving**.
Battery is flat.

That is what real eco cars do.
They pause every now and then,
they respect the **environment**.

And we need to walk.
What's more eco than that?

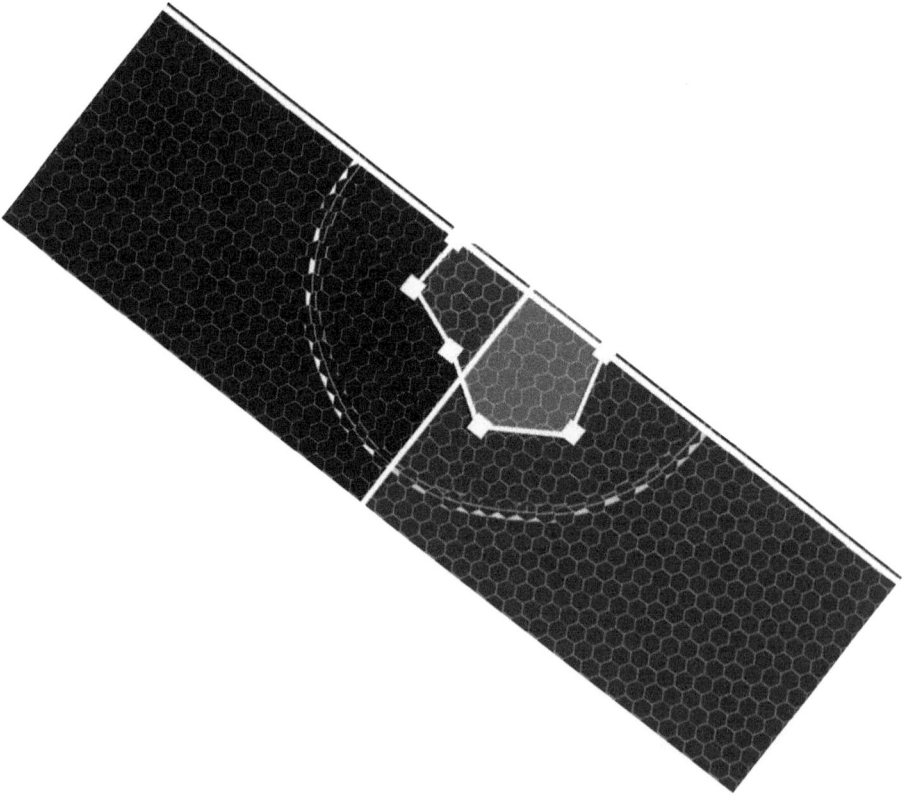

Informal timetable,
date for disclosure,
6 weeks.

Witness statements,
before and after,
evi dence.

Neuro log,
neuro otol,
neuro psych.

Psycho log,
physio ther,
audio lo.

Thera psy,
psychi tra,
occu health.

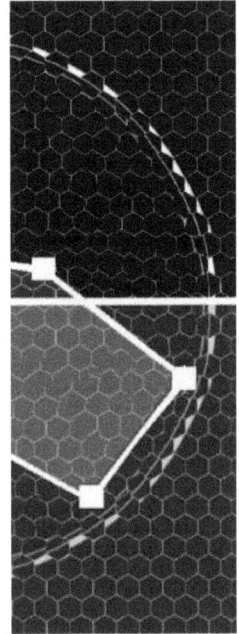

Medical journey all in line.

Dolce Vita
in a close
of Hastings town.

Geraniums' furniture
in rose display
with toxic green.

Purple bells
are climbing up
the Mi-mo-sa.

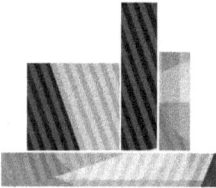

Warmer feel
in cork blocks
of salvia gray.

Growing grass
as it's rolling
in the stones.
Dark red acer
calling myrtus
up the hill.

Hastings town standing still in moving clouds.

Spoon_76 : A Heart Balloon

An epic sphere in the air with the form of a heart.

Not sure if it's broken or if it's still very intact.

As it turns, we can see that there is a red blood track.

Dripping fluid on the clouds, red on white as a con-trast.

As it turns, two cracked veins we clearly see.

Blood is flooding all the sky, as it's spraying a deadly dye.

Hearts can crack and go, in a moment with no stop.

I am sorry if I caused the spill, if it helps, there was no will.

The heart balloon can still reach the moon.

Believe it, you are free.

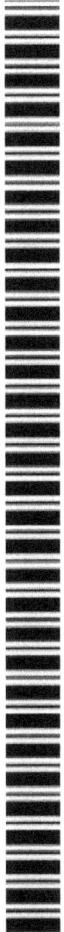

Our champions are going for gold.

1

spoon

at

a

time.

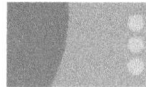

Void.

Spoon_79 : Thanks Off

Thanks Off
to **the** painful ones.

Thanks Off
to the **moments** of despair.

Thanks Off
to that liberation never coming.

Thanks Off
to the dark shadow **matters**.

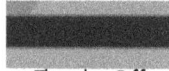

Thanks Off
to every single heavy punch.

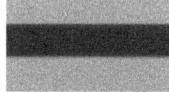

Thanks Off
to that pressing never stopping.

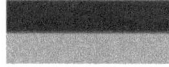

Thanks Off
for asking but not caring.

Thanks Off
and
Duck You!

Pulling-off the impossible
is an appetizer
of what's to come.

Believe in yourself,
weather-proofed
in accepting limits.

Limits that once seen
can slowly change
as **you** commit.

Be thankful. Be humble. Be precise.

Recognise your spoons,
and protect them
every single day.

Keep your eyes inside your system,
don't rush,
take your time.

And remember that even on the toughest day,
you **will** do it in your unique way.

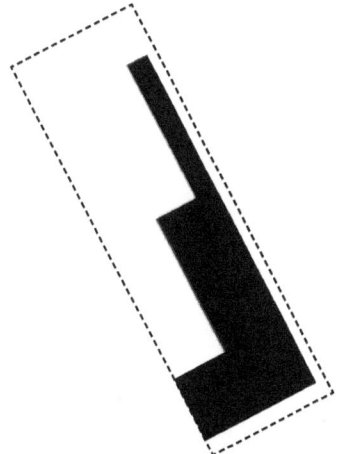

www.ingramcontent.com/pod-product-compliance
Lightning Source LLC
Chambersburg PA
CBHW042122190326
41519CB00031B/7581